Intermittent Fasting for Beginners

The Ultimate Guide to Effortless Weight Loss and Optimal Health

Sarah Carsen

Intermittent Fasting for Beginners

Copyright 2024 © Sarah Carsen

ALL RIGHTS RESERVED

No part of this publication may be reproduced, stored in a retrieval system, or transmitted, in any form or by any means, electronic, mechanical, photocopying, recording or otherwise, without the express written permission of the author.

DISCLAIMER

No part of this publication may be reproduced, stored in a retrieval system, or transmitted, in any form or by any means, electronic, mechanical, photocopying, recording or otherwise, without the express written permission of the author.

Table of Contents

Appendix   66

About the Author   81

Introduction

In the face of today's challenges, maintaining a balanced and healthy lifestyle might appear to be an impossible task. Meet Barbara, a dedicated woman in her mid-40s who previously became locked in a cycle of fad diets and fleeting fitness trends. She who was struggling with excess weight and poor health, felt trapped in a body that no longer felt like her own.

However, in the midst of her anguish and despair, she discovered a solution that would transform her life: *intermittent fasting*.

Barbara, felt empowered and liberated as she began her adventure of intermittent fasting. With each passing day, she felt the weight of her old habits shift, giving way to a fresh vigor and mental clarity.

She not only lost the pounds that had been bothering her for years, but she also regained control of her health and well-being thanks to the simple yet profound practice of intermittent fasting. Her story is one of both physical and inner strength, demonstrating the life-changing effects of a sustainable approach to health.

In *"Intermittent Fasting for Beginners: The Ultimate Guide to Effortless Weight Loss and Optimal Health,"* I encourage you to follow Barbara's example and start your own road to wellbeing. Whether you're a busy professional juggling work and family responsibilities, a new mom dealing with the obstacles of postpartum weight loss, or just looking for a fresh start on the path to improved health, this book is your comprehensive guide to success.

These pages will teach you all you need to know about intermittent fasting and how to maximize its benefits. From demystifying the science behind this potent nutritional strategy to giving practical recommendations for smoothly integrating fasting protocols into your everyday routine, this guide has you covered.

With customized meal plans, delectable recipes, and expert advice from the me, you'll discover how to use intermittent fasting to lose weight easily, improve your health, and reinvigorate your life.

So, are you ready to rewrite your story and start on a path to a better, happier yourself? Allow *"Intermittent Fasting for Beginners"* to be your reliable guide on the way to long-term wellbeing.

Say goodbye to fad diets and short solutions and adopt a long-term strategy that enables you to take control of your health and alter your life from the inside out. Your adventure begins here; let's make it memorable!

CHAPTER 1

Decoding Intermittent Fasting

1.1 What is Intermittent Fasting?

Intermittent fasting is an eating pattern in which individuals alternate between eating and fasting. Instead of focusing exclusively on what meals to consume or avoid, intermittent fasting emphasizes when to eat. It entails alternating between times of eating and fasting in order to provide a variety of health advantages, including weight loss, improved metabolic health, and increased longevity. This method of eating has grown popularity in recent years because to its simplicity, adaptability, and possible health advantages.

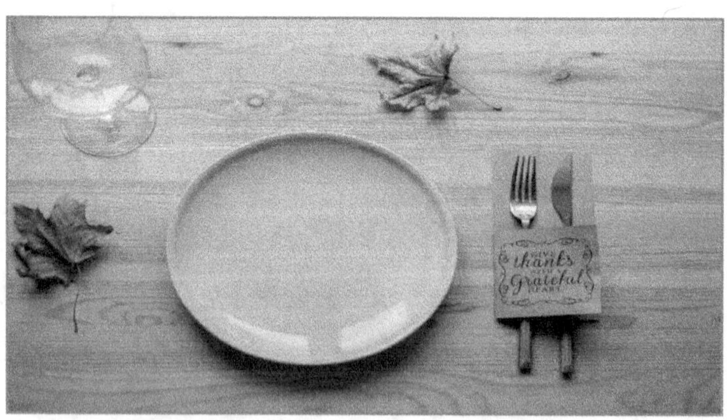

1.2 History and Evolution of Intermittent Fasting

Intermittent fasting, while fashionable in recent years, has a long history extending back millennia. Its origins may be traced back to ancient civilizations, where fasting was practiced for religious, spiritual, and cultural purposes. The ancient Greeks felt that fasting on occasion was beneficial to physical and mental health, and several religious traditions, including Christianity, Judaism, and Islam, include fasting into their practices.

One of the first known cases of intermittent fasting dates back to ancient Greece, when Pythagoras, the Greek philosopher, supposedly called for periodic fasting as a method of increasing health and life. Seneca, a Stoic philosopher from ancient Rome, embraced intermittent fasting as a kind of self-discipline and moderation.

Fasting has historically been associated with a variety of cultural and religious rituals. For example, the Islamic practice of Ramadan entails fasting from sunrise to sunset for a month, whereas the Christian tradition of Lent includes fasting and abstaining from particular meals in the run-up to Easter.

In the early twentieth century, scientists began to investigate the physiological consequences of fasting on health. Dr. Luigi Cornaro, an Italian aristocrat from the 15th century, was a well-known person in this subject.

Cornaro notably underwent calorie restriction and intermittent fasting, which he documented in his book *"Discourses on the Sober Life."*

In recent years, intermittent fasting has received scientific interest due to its possible health advantages. In the twentieth century, researchers like as Drs. Nathan Pritikin and Roy Walford investigated the effects of calorie restriction and intermittent fasting on longevity and disease prevention.

Intermittent fasting is becoming a popular dietary practice, with millions of individuals worldwide following various fasting regimens for weight loss, improved metabolic health, and other health advantages. While intermittent fasting is still evolving, its rich history underlines its ongoing appeal as a time-honored practice with far-reaching implications for human health and wellness.

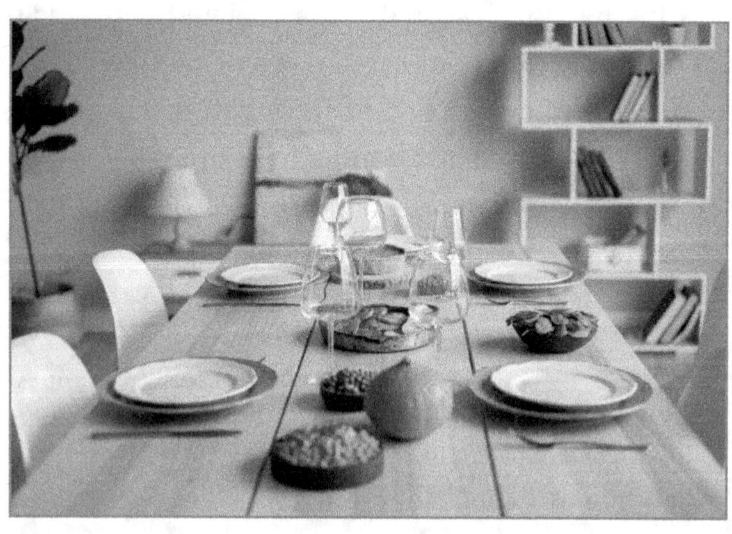

1.3 How Intermittent Fasting Works

Intermittent fasting works on the idea of alternating between eating and fasting, altering numerous physiological processes in the body to enhance health and well-being. When a person engages in intermittent fasting, many important mechanisms work together to create the desired results.

One of the most important aspects of intermittent fasting is how it affects insulin levels and sensitivity. During fasting, the body's insulin levels drop, allowing stored glucose to be mobilized and utilized as energy. This lowers blood sugar levels and gradually increases insulin sensitivity, lowering the risk of insulin resistance and type 2 diabetes.

Additionally, intermittent fasting causes a metabolic shift from glucose to fat metabolism. When the body does not get a consistent supply of glucose from meals, it begins to break down stored fat for energy via a process known as lipolysis. This leads in the formation of ketone bodies, which act as an alternate fuel source for cells, notably those in the brain and muscles.

This metabolic condition, known as ketosis, promotes fat burning and may aid in weight reduction and improved body composition.

Intermittent fasting also encourages autophagy, a cellular repair mechanism that occurs in response to starvation and food deficiency. During fasting, cells clean themselves by eliminating damaged or malfunctioning components and recycling them for energy.

Autophagy is critical for cellular health and longevity, helping to preserve cellular integrity and function while lowering the risk of age-related illnesses.

Furthermore, intermittent fasting has been demonstrated to influence a variety of hormones and signaling pathways involved in metabolism, inflammation, and stress response.

Fasting, for example, enhances the synthesis of growth hormone, which helps to maintain muscle mass and promotes fat reduction. It also stimulates pathways linked to lifespan and cellular resilience, which improves the body's capacity to adapt to external challenges and sustain peak performance.

As a whole, intermittent fasting works by utilizing the body's natural mechanisms to improve metabolic health, weight reduction, and cellular repair.

Individuals may optimize their physiology and gain the multiple benefits of this nutritional strategy by carefully scheduling their eating and fasting times.

CHAPTER 2

Choosing Your Fasting Window

2.1 16/8 Method: The Popular Time-Restricted Eating Approach

The 16/8 method, often known as the 16-hour fast or time-restricted eating, is a popular and extensively performed kind of intermittent fasting. It entails cycling between eating and fasting intervals throughout the day, with individuals fasting for 16 hours and limiting their eating window to 8 hours each day. This method has gained popularity due to its simplicity, adaptability, and possible health advantages.

The 16/8 method usually includes foregoing breakfast and postponing the first meal of the day until later in the morning or early afternoon.

For example, someone using this strategy would take their first meal around midday and then consume all of their calories within an 8-hour period, concluding by 8 p.m. They would then fast for the remaining 16 hours until the next day's eating window opened.

The 16/8 method's appeal stems mostly from its simplicity. Compared to more sophisticated fasting protocols like alternate day fasting or the 5:2 diet, the 16/8 approach is comparatively simple to start and follow on a daily basis. It does not need calorie tracking or careful meal preparation, making it suitable for a wide spectrum of people.

Furthermore, the 16/8 technique provides flexibility, allowing people to tailor their eating schedule to their lifestyle and interests. Some people like to eat earlier in the day, while others eat later.

This adaptability makes intermittent fasting simpler to integrate into everyday routines while accommodating social gatherings or work schedules.

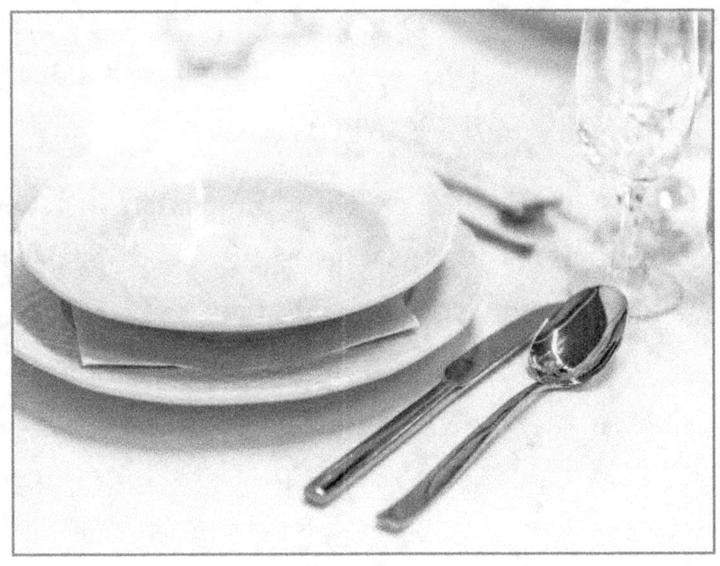

2.2 5:2 Diet: Incorporating Fasting Days into Your Week

The 5:2 diet is a type of intermittent fasting in which you eat normally five days a week and limit your calorie intake to 500-600 calories on the other two days. Fasting days can be consecutive or non-consecutive, providing flexibility in implementation.

On fasting days, people usually eat short meals or snacks that are low in calories, such vegetables, fruits, lean meats, and soup. The objective is to dramatically reduce calorie consumption while maintaining critical nutrients for general health.

One of the 5:2 diet's main advantages is its flexibility. Unlike other types of intermittent fasting, which require daily fasting or strict meal scheduling, the 5:2 diet allows people to eat regularly most days of the week, making it simpler to stick to in the long run.

This adaptability also makes it simpler to include into social gatherings or special occasions, as fasting days may be tailored to individual schedules.

2.3 Alternate Day Fasting: A Flexible Fasting Routine

Alternate day fasting is an intermittent fasting method in which you alternate between days of usual eating and days of fasting. On fasting days, people dramatically restrict their calorie intake or refrain from meals entirely, but on non-fasting days, they eat regularly.

This adaptable fasting routine is a simple yet effective strategy to encourage weight reduction, improve metabolic health, and boost overall well-being.

One of the primary advantages of alternate day fasting is its versatility. Unlike other intermittent fasting approaches that demand daily fasting or specified meal timing, alternate day fasting allows people to fast on the days that work best for them based on their schedule and preferences.

This flexibility makes it simpler to follow in the long run and may be tailored to different lifestyles and dietary choices.

However, alternate day fasting may not be appropriate for everyone. Some people may find it difficult to stick to a fasting schedule on alternate days, while others may experience undesirable side effects such as hunger, weariness, or irritation. Before beginning any fasting routine, pay close attention to your body and speak with a healthcare practitioner, especially if you have underlying health concerns or are taking drugs.

2.4 OMAD (One Meal a Day): Simplifying Your Eating Window

OMAD, or One Meal a Day, is a type of intermittent fasting in which all daily calories are consumed during a single meal window that lasts around one hour. This strategy greatly simplifies the eating window, allowing people to fast for the most of the day and have only one large meal.

One of the primary benefits of OMAD is that it's simple. Unlike other intermittent fasting methods, which divide the day into particular fasting and eating times, OMAD streamlines the process by combining all food consumption into a single meal.

This might be especially appealing to individuals who don't want to spend time planning and cooking many meals during the day.

Furthermore, OMAD allows for greater meal time flexibility. While some people choose to have their OMAD meals at the same time every day, others may opt to change up their meal times based on their schedule or preferences.

This flexibility enables people to customize OMAD to meet their lifestyle and accommodate social activities or job requirements.

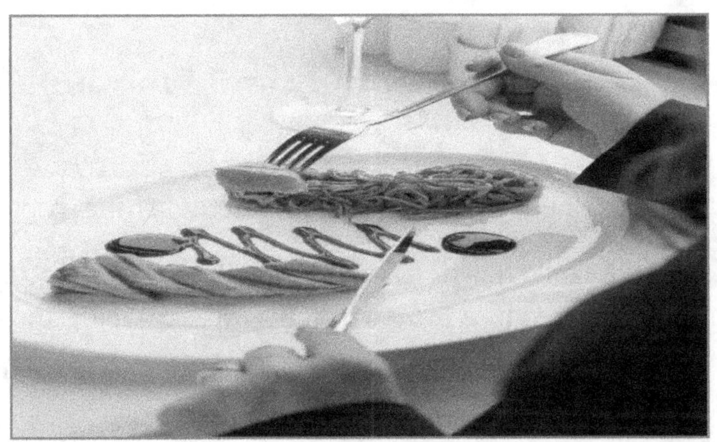

CHAPTER 3

Getting Started with Intermittent Fasting

3.1 Preparing Mentally and Emotionally

Before beginning any intermittent fasting program, you must first prepare psychologically and emotionally. While intermittent fasting can provide several health advantages, success and long-term viability require the correct mentality and emotional preparation.

One of the first stages in psychologically and emotionally preparing for intermittent fasting is to establish reasonable expectations. Understand that intermittent fasting is neither a quick fix nor a one-size-fits-all approach.

For one to witness long-term outcomes, patience, consistency, and perseverance are required. Recognize that there may be obstacles along the path, but with endurance and drive, you will overcome them.

Learning more about intermittent fasting might also help you psychologically and emotionally prepare for the trip ahead. Discover the many fasting strategies, how they operate, and the possible advantages and drawbacks connected with each.

Understanding intermittent fasting will help reduce your concerns and anxiety, allowing you to make educated decisions regarding your fasting schedule.

Another key part of mental and emotional preparation is developing a good attitude. Approach intermittent fasting with inquiry, openness, and optimism. Focus on the possible benefits of fasting, such as weight loss, better metabolic health, higher energy, and mental clarity.

Visualize yourself attaining your health and wellness objectives through intermittent fasting, and use this as incentive to stick to your fasting schedule.

During intermittent fasting, you should also listen to your body and respect your hunger cues. Pay attention to how you feel physically, intellectually, and emotionally during the fasting time.

If you're feeling extreme hunger, exhaustion, or other discomfort, don't be afraid to change your fasting schedule or get advice from a healthcare practitioner or nutrition expert.

Finally, during your intermittent fasting journey, be nice and kind to yourself. Understand that there will be ups and downs, and it is OK to experience setbacks along the path. Be kind with yourself and celebrate your accomplishments, no matter how little.

Remember that intermittent fasting is only one component of a healthy lifestyle, and you should also prioritize your entire well-being and self-care.

3.2 Clearing Common Misconceptions

Intermittent fasting has been popular in recent years as a dietary strategy for weight reduction and increased health. However, as it has grown in popularity, intermittent fasting has given birth to a number of myths and misunderstandings.

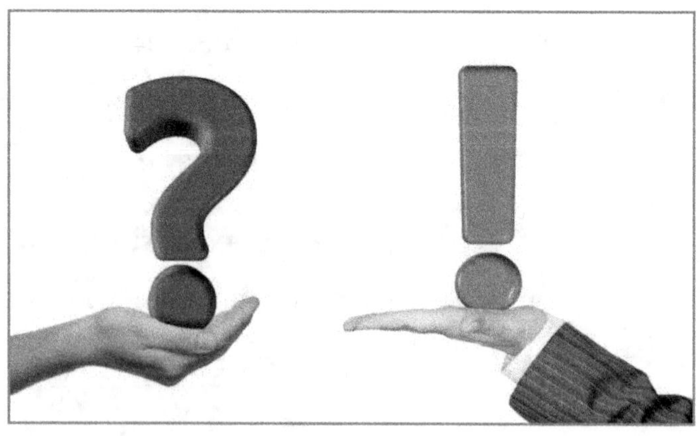

It is critical to clarify these myths so that people have correct information about intermittent fasting and may make educated decisions about implementing it into their lives.

One prevalent misperception regarding intermittent fasting is that it needs stringent calorie tracking or significant dietary restriction. While some types of intermittent fasting, such as the 5:2 diet or alternate day fasting, limit calorie intake during fasting periods, others, such as the 16/8 technique or OMAD (One Meal a Day), restrict eating schedule rather than amount.

Intermittent fasting provides for greater flexibility in meal choices and portion amounts during eating windows, making it a more sustainable alternative to typical calorie-restricted diets.

Another misunderstanding regarding intermittent fasting is that it causes muscle loss and decreases metabolism. Intermittent fasting, when paired with resistance exercise, has been shown to retain muscle mass and even enhance muscular development.

Additionally, intermittent fasting has been proven to offer metabolic advantages, such as enhancing insulin sensitivity and boosting fat reduction, which can assist improve overall metabolic health.

There is also a misperception that intermittent fasting is only appropriate for specific groups, such as young, healthy individuals. In actuality, intermittent fasting may be tailored to a variety of people, including older folks, those with chronic health concerns, and even sports.

Individuals with underlying health concerns or unique nutritional demands should check with a healthcare provider before beginning an intermittent fasting plan.

Furthermore, intermittent fasting is frequently misconstrued as a *"quick fix"* or short-term weight loss option. Intermittent fasting can provide quick initial weight reduction owing to changes in water weight and glycogen storage, but long-term weight loss needs commitment to healthy eating habits and lifestyle improvements.

Intermittent fasting should be seen as part of a holistic health and wellness strategy that includes balanced eating, frequent physical exercise, and appropriate sleep.

There is also a misperception that intermittent fasting equates to starvation or eating problems. While both entail periods of dietary restriction, intermittent fasting differs significantly from starvation and eating disorders.

Intermittent fasting is an organized and regulated approach to eating that promotes health and well-being, whereas starvation and eating disorders are characterized by harmful food and body image views. Intermittent fasting should be approached with a healthy mentality, with a focus on feeding the body rather than reducing food intake for weight reduction.

3.3 Setting Realistic Expectations

Setting reasonable expectations is critical when starting an intermittent fasting adventure. While intermittent fasting has various health benefits, it is critical to approach it with a clear awareness of what it can and cannot do.

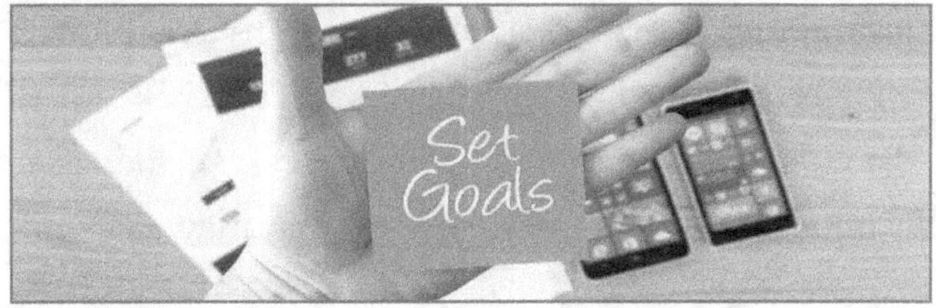

First and first, it's critical to understand that intermittent fasting is neither a quick cure or a one-size-fits-all answer to weight reduction or health improvement. While some people lose weight quickly with intermittent fasting, long-term outcomes need time, consistency, and patience.

It is critical to set realistic objectives and recognize that development might be sluggish and vary from person to person.

Furthermore, intermittent fasting is not a quick fix for many health concerns.

While it can help with weight reduction, metabolic health, and general well-being, it is only one part of a holistic approach to health and wellbeing.

To get the most advantages from intermittent fasting, it's critical to prioritize other parts of a healthy lifestyle, such as balanced eating, frequent physical activity, appropriate sleep, and stress management.

Furthermore, it is vital to recognize that intermittent fasting may not be appropriate for everyone. Individuals with certain medical concerns, such as diabetes, eating disorders, or hormonal imbalances, should exercise caution or avoid intermittent fasting entirely.

It is critical to check with a healthcare practitioner before beginning an intermittent fasting routine, especially if you have underlying health concerns or are taking drugs.

Also, intermittent fasting may provide problems and potential negative effects, particularly during the first adjustment period.

Common side effects include hunger, exhaustion, irritability, and trouble focusing. Listen to your body, heed your hunger cues, and make any necessary changes to your fasting schedule or nutritional consumption.

If you are experiencing chronic or severe adverse effects, see a healthcare physician or nutrition specialist.

CHAPTER 4

Crafting Your Personalized Meal Plans

4.1 Understanding Nutrient-Rich Foods

Understanding nutrient-dense foods is critical for sustaining good health and well-being, especially when using dietary techniques such as intermittent fasting.

Nutrient-dense foods have a high concentration of important nutrients compared to their calorie level. Vitamins, minerals, antioxidants, fiber, and healthy fats are all essential nutrients that support numerous biological activities and promote overall health.

Fruits and vegetables are nutrient-dense foods. These colorful plant foods are high in vitamins, minerals, and antioxidants, which boost the immune system, defend against chronic illnesses, and improve general health. Include a variety of fruits and vegetables in your diet, preferably in different hues, to provide a varied spectrum of nutrients.

Whole grains are an excellent source of nutrients, including complex carbs, fiber, vitamins, and minerals. Choose whole grains such as brown rice, quinoa, oats, and barley, which contain more minerals and fiber than refined grains like white rice or white bread. Whole grains can help control blood sugar levels, improve digestive health, and give steady energy throughout the day.

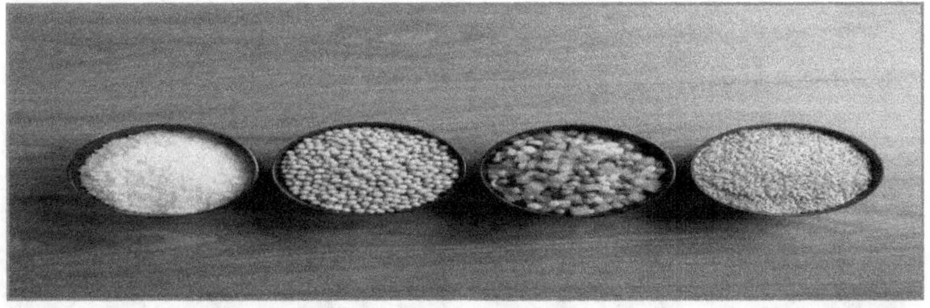

Lean proteins are necessary for tissue growth and repair, muscular health, and metabolic regulation. Choose lean protein sources including chicken, fish, tofu, beans, lentils, and low-fat dairy products. These foods include high-quality protein as well as important amino acids, vitamins, and minerals, but with no extra saturated fat or added sugar.

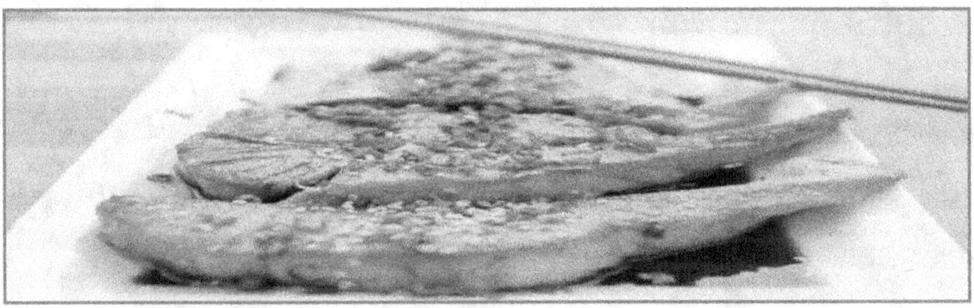

Healthy fats are another vital component of a nutrient-dense diet, since they contain necessary fatty acids that promote brain health, hormone synthesis, and cell functionality. Avocados, almonds, seeds, olive oil, and fatty seafood such as salmon and sardines are also good sources of healthful fat.

These meals contain monounsaturated and polyunsaturated fats that are beneficial to the heart, as well as vitamins and antioxidants.

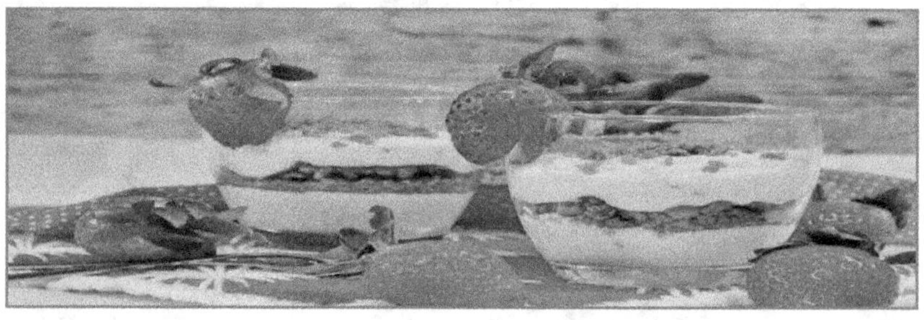

Dairy products are high in calcium, vitamin D, and other important minerals that promote bone health, muscular function, and general well-being. Choose low-fat or non-fat dairy products like milk, yogurt, and cheese to reduce your saturated fat consumption while still reaping nutritional advantages.

Incorporating a variety of nutrient-rich foods into your diet is critical for maintaining overall health and well-being, especially if you practice intermittent fasting. While intermittent fasting can provide several health advantages, it is critical to prioritize nutrient-dense meals during eating windows to ensure that your body obtains the necessary resources to function properly.

When preparing meals during eating windows, aim for a balance of macronutrients (carbohydrates, protein, and fats) and micronutrients (vitamins, minerals). To guarantee a well-rounded and nutrient-dense diet, eat a variety of fruits and vegetables, whole grains, lean meats, healthy fats, and dairy products.

It is also critical to remain hydrated while eating food by drinking enough of water and other hydrating liquids. Avoid sugary beverages and excessive caffeine, which can cause dehydration and disturb energy levels.

4.2 Designing Balanced Meals for Fasting Periods

Designing balanced meals for fasting periods is critical to ensuring that your body obtains enough nutrients and energy to support you throughout the fasting time.

While fasting limits the amount of time available for eating, it is still vital to prioritize nutrient-dense foods, as earlier stated, and prepare meals that contain a variety of macronutrients (carbohydrates, protein, and fats) as well as necessary vitamins and minerals. Here's a tip on creating balanced meals during fasting periods:

1.*Include Protein:* Protein is required to maintain muscle growth, enhance immunological function, and promote satiety. Include lean protein in your meals, such as chicken, fish, tofu, beans, lentils, eggs, or Greek yogurt. Protein-rich meals might help you feel full and satisfied during your fasting phase.

2.*Include Healthy Fats:* Healthy fats are essential for delivering long-lasting energy, maintaining brain function, and absorbing fat-soluble vitamins. Avocados, almonds, seeds, olive oil, and fatty seafood such as salmon or sardines may all provide healthy fats in your diet. These meals can help you feel satiated while also providing critical nutrients during fasting times.

3.*Choose Complex carbs:* Complex carbs give a consistent source of energy and aid in blood sugar control. Choose whole grains such brown rice, quinoa, oats, barley, and whole wheat bread. Incorporating complex carbs into your meals will help you stay energized and reduce blood sugar spikes and crashes when fasting.

4.*Include Fiber-Rich Foods:* Fiber is beneficial to digestive health, encouraging fullness, and managing blood sugar levels. Include fiber-rich items in your diet, such as fruits, vegetables, legumes, and whole grains. These meals can help you feel full and satisfied while also supplying critical nutrients and promoting overall health.

5.*Prioritize Nutrient-Dense meals:* Choose nutrient-dense meals that include a diverse variety of vitamins, minerals, and antioxidants. Include a variety of colored fruits and vegetables in your meals to ensure you obtain a wide range of nutrients.

In addition, include calcium, iron, vitamin D, and other necessary nutrients to promote general health and well-being.

6.*Stay Hydrated:* During fasting times, consume lots of water and other hydrating liquids. Drink at least 8-10 glasses of water every day, and consider adding herbal teas or infused water for extra taste and hydration. Staying hydrated can help avoid dehydration, aid digestion, and boost general health during fasting times.

7.*Mindful Eating:* During fasting times, focus on your body's hunger and fullness indicators. Eat gently, relishing each bite, and be aware of how your body feels during the meal. This can help you avoid overeating and feel more satisfied with your meals.

8.Plan Ahead: Plan your meals and snacks ahead of time to ensure that you have a variety of alternatives accessible during fasts. To prevent grabbing for convenience foods or harmful snacks, plan your meals ahead of time, portion out snacks, and keep healthy alternatives on hand.

Designing balanced meals during fasting times ensures that your body obtains the nutrition and energy it requires to promote general health and well-being.

4.3 Sample Meal Plans for Different Fasting Windows

Creating sample meal plans for different fasting windows can help individuals navigate their intermittent fasting journey effectively. These meal plans provide guidance on what to eat during eating windows to ensure balanced nutrition, promote satiety, and support overall health and well-being.

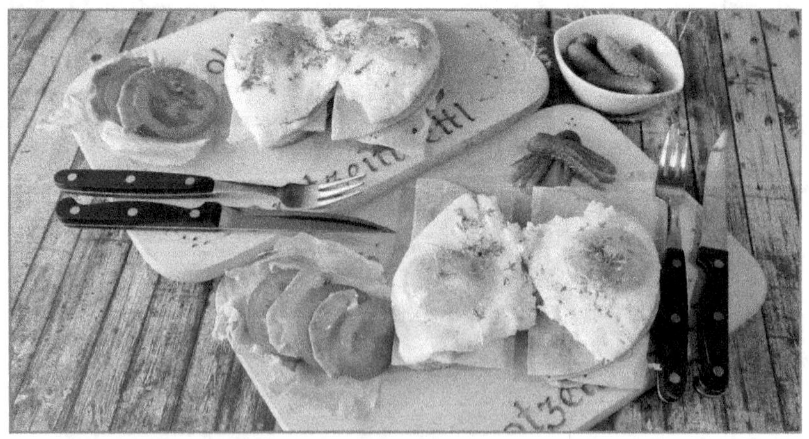

Below are sample meal plans for three common fasting windows: 16/8 method, 5:2 diet, and OMAD (One Meal a Day).

16/8 Method Meal Plan:

The 16/8 method involves fasting for 16 hours and eating within an 8-hour window each day. Here's a sample meal plan for a day following the 16/8 method:

(Day 1)

Eating Window: 12:00 pm - 8:00 pm

12:00 pm (Meal 1):

- Grilled chicken breast

- Quinoa salad with mixed vegetables (bell peppers, cucumber, cherry tomatoes)

- Balsamic vinaigrette dressing

- 1 small apple

3:00 pm (Snack):

- Greek yogurt with sliced almonds and berries

6:00 pm (Meal 2):

- Baked salmon fillet

- Steamed broccoli

- Brown rice

- Mixed green salad with olive oil and lemon dressing

8:00 pm (Snack):

- Handful of mixed nuts (almonds, walnuts, pistachios)

16/8 Method Meal Plan (Day 2):

Eating Window: 10:00 am - 6:00 pm

10:00 am (Meal 1):

- Overnight oats made with rolled oats, almond milk, chia seeds, sliced banana, and a drizzle of honey

- Hard-boiled egg on the side

1:00 pm (Meal 2):

- Turkey and avocado wrap made with whole wheat tortilla, sliced turkey breast, avocado, lettuce, tomato, and mustard

- Carrot sticks with hummus

4:00 pm (Snack):

- Greek yogurt parfait with layers of Greek yogurt, mixed berries, and granola

6:00 pm (Meal 3):

- Grilled shrimp skewers with bell peppers, onions, and pineapple

- Quinoa pilaf with mixed herbs

- Steamed asparagus with lemon zest

This meal plan provides a variety of nutrient-dense foods to support overall health and well-being throughout the eating window.

5:2 Diet Meal Plan:

The 5:2 diet involves eating normally for five days of the week and restricting calorie intake to around 500-600 calories on the remaining two days. Here's a sample meal plan for a fasting day following the 5:2 diet:

Fasting Day (Day 1):

Breakfast (150 calories):

- 1 boiled egg

- 1 slice of whole wheat toast

Lunch (250 calories):

- Mixed green salad with cherry tomatoes, cucumber, and balsamic vinaigrette dressing

- 3 oz grilled chicken breast

Dinner (200 calories):

- Steamed vegetables (broccoli, carrots, cauliflower)

- 1/2 cup cooked quinoa

5:2 Diet Meal Plan:

Fasting Day (Day 2):

Breakfast (150 calories):

- Spinach and feta egg muffins (2 muffins)

Lunch (250 calories):

- Tomato and basil soup (1 cup)

- Mixed green salad with cucumber, bell peppers, and balsamic vinaigrette dressing

Dinner (200 calories):

- Baked salmon fillet (3 oz)

- Steamed broccoli (1 cup)

This meal plan offers around 600 calories for a fasting day on the 5:2 diet, with a focus on protein-rich foods and fiber-rich vegetables to promote satiety despite the calorie restriction.

OMAD (One Meal a Day) Meal Plan:

The OMAD (One Meal a Day) method involves consuming all daily calories within a single meal window, typically lasting around one hour.

Here's a sample meal plan for a day following the OMAD method:

Eating Window: 6:00 pm - 7:00 pm

6:00 pm (Meal) Day 1:

- Grilled steak with roasted vegetables (bell peppers, zucchini, onions)

- Baked sweet potato

- Mixed green salad with avocado, feta cheese, and balsamic vinaigrette dressing

- 1 small piece of dark chocolate for dessert

Meal Plan (Day 2):

Eating Window: 5:30 pm - 6:30 pm

5:30 pm (Meal):

- Lentil and vegetable curry served over brown rice

- Mixed green salad with cherry tomatoes, cucumber, and lemon vinaigrette dressing

- Roasted sweet potato wedges

- Sliced mango for dessert

This meal plan provides a balance of plant-based protein, complex carbohydrates, fiber, and essential nutrients within a single meal window, supporting overall health and well-being despite consuming all daily calories in one sitting.

CHAPTER 5

Troubleshooting Common Challenges

5.1 Overcoming Hunger Pangs

Overcoming hunger pangs is a common challenge when practicing intermittent fasting, but there are strategies you can employ to manage hunger and stay on track with your fasting regimen.

One effective way to overcome hunger pangs during fasting periods is to stay hydrated by drinking plenty of water throughout the day. Sometimes, feelings of hunger can be mistaken for dehydration, so staying hydrated can help curb cravings and keep you feeling full.

In addition, consuming beverages like herbal tea or black coffee can help suppress appetite and provide a temporary sense of fullness without breaking your fast. Just be mindful of adding sugar or cream to your drinks, as this can add unnecessary calories and potentially disrupt the fasting state.

Another strategy for managing hunger pangs is to distract yourself with activities or tasks that keep your mind occupied. Engaging in activities like reading, going for a walk, or practicing mindfulness exercises can help take your focus away from food and reduce feelings of hunger.

Adding high-fiber foods into your meals can also help keep you feeling full for longer periods. Fiber-rich foods like fruits, vegetables, whole grains, and legumes take longer to digest, which can help control hunger and prevent overeating during eating windows.

Furthermore, paying attention to meal timing and composition can help minimize hunger pangs during fasting periods. Try to schedule your meals strategically, so you're eating meals that are satisfying and filling, and include a balance of protein, healthy fats, and complex carbohydrates to help stabilize blood sugar levels and promote satiety.

Lastly, it's essential to listen to your body and honor your hunger cues while practicing intermittent fasting. If you're experiencing persistent or severe hunger pangs, it may be a sign that you need to adjust your fasting schedule or meal composition to better meet your body's needs.

By incorporating these strategies into your fasting routine, you can effectively manage hunger and stay on track with your health and wellness goals.

5.2 Dealing with Social Situations and Dining Out

Navigating social situations and dining out while practicing intermittent fasting can present challenges, but with some planning and flexibility, it's possible to enjoy social events without derailing your fasting goals.

One approach to dealing with social situations is to communicate your dietary preferences or fasting regimen with friends and family beforehand. Letting them know about your fasting schedule can help manage expectations and reduce pressure to eat during social gatherings. Most people will be understanding and supportive of your choices.

When dining out, it's helpful to research restaurant menus ahead of time and choose options that align with your fasting goals. Look for dishes that are rich in protein, vegetables, and healthy fats, which can help keep you feeling full and satisfied during the fasting window.

Additionally, consider asking for modifications to accommodate your dietary preferences, such as swapping out high-calorie sides for steamed vegetables or opting for dressings and sauces on the side.

If you're attending a social event where food will be served, focus on enjoying the company of others rather than solely on the food. Engage in conversations, participate in activities, and find other ways to connect with those around you that don't revolve around eating. Bringing a non-caloric beverage like water or herbal tea can also help occupy your hands and prevent mindless snacking.

Another strategy for managing social situations and dining out is to practice mindfulness and intuitive eating. Pay attention to your body's hunger and fullness cues, and eat only when you're truly hungry. Avoid mindless eating or overindulging out of social pressure, and listen to your body's signals to guide your food choices.

It's also important to give yourself permission to enjoy special occasions and occasional indulgences without guilt. If you choose to break your fast or deviate from your usual eating pattern during a social event, remind yourself that it's okay and that one meal or snack won't undo all of your progress. The key is to maintain balance and consistency over the long term.

5.3 Combating Fatigue and Low Energy

Combatting fatigue and low energy levels while practicing intermittent fasting is essential for maintaining overall well-being and productivity. Here are some strategies to help boost energy levels and combat fatigue during fasting periods:

Firstly, ensure that you're staying hydrated by drinking plenty of water throughout the day, like earlier stated. Dehydration can contribute to feelings of fatigue, so it's crucial to replenish fluids regularly, especially during fasting periods. Herbal teas and electrolyte-rich beverages can also help support hydration and boost energy levels.

Consuming nutrient-dense foods during eating windows can help provide sustained energy throughout the day. Focus on incorporating a balance of protein, healthy fats, complex carbohydrates, and fiber-rich foods into your meals to help stabilize blood sugar levels and prevent energy crashes. Include foods like lean meats, fish, eggs, nuts, seeds, whole grains, fruits, and vegetables to support overall energy levels.

Prioritize adequate rest and sleep to combat fatigue and support overall well-being. Aim for 7-9 hours of quality sleep per night and establish a consistent sleep schedule to regulate your body's internal clock. Create a relaxing bedtime routine, limit screen time before bed, and create a comfortable sleep environment to promote restful sleep.

Integrate regular physical activity into your routine to help boost energy levels and combat fatigue. Engage in activities you enjoy, such as walking, jogging, yoga, or strength training, to help increase blood flow, improve mood, and boost energy levels. Aim for at least 30 minutes of moderate-intensity exercise most days of the week to reap the benefits of physical activity.

Practice stress management techniques like mindfulness, meditation, deep breathing exercises, or progressive muscle relaxation to help reduce stress levels and combat fatigue. Chronic stress can contribute to feelings of fatigue and low energy, so it's essential to prioritize relaxation and self-care practices to support overall well-being.

Finally, as stated constantly, listen to your body and honor your hunger and fullness cues during fasting periods. If you're experiencing excessive fatigue or low energy levels, it may be a sign that you need to adjust your fasting schedule or meal composition to better meet your body's needs. Consider experimenting with different fasting protocols, meal timing, or nutrient ratios to find what works best for you.

5.4 Adjusting Your Fasting Routine for Your Lifestyle

Adjusting your fasting routine to suit your lifestyle is key to ensuring long-term adherence and success with intermittent fasting. Here are some strategies for tailoring your fasting regimen to fit your individual needs and preferences:

1. *Flexible Fasting Windows:* Experiment with different fasting windows to find what works best for your lifestyle. While some people prefer a standard 16/8 fasting window (fasting for 16 hours and eating within an 8-hour window), others may find it more manageable to shorten or lengthen their fasting periods based on their schedule and preferences. Consider factors like work hours, social commitments, and personal preferences when determining your fasting window.

2. *Meal Timing:* Adjust the timing of your meals to align with your daily routine and energy needs. If you're more active in the morning, consider shifting your eating window earlier in the day to fuel your activities. Alternatively, if you prefer larger meals in the evening or have social obligations that revolve around dinner, adjust your fasting window accordingly.

3. Fasting Frequency: Experiment with different fasting frequencies to find a schedule that fits your lifestyle and goals. Some people may thrive on a daily fasting schedule, while others may prefer intermittent fasting on alternate days or a few times per week. Consider your level of hunger, energy levels, and overall well-being when determining how often to incorporate fasting into your routine.

4. Social Considerations: Plan ahead for social events and gatherings to ensure that you can participate while still adhering to your fasting regimen. Communicate your dietary preferences or fasting schedule with friends and family, and consider strategies like adjusting your fasting window or making mindful food choices while dining out.

5. Listen to Your Body: Pay attention to how your body responds to different fasting protocols and adjust your routine accordingly. If you're experiencing excessive hunger, fatigue, or other negative side effects, it may be a sign that you need to modify your fasting schedule or meal composition. Listen to your body's cues and make changes as needed to support your overall health and well-being.

CHAPTER 6

Fine-Tuning Your Intermittent Fasting Journey

6.1 Listening to Your Body's Signals

Listening to your body's signals is crucial when practicing intermittent fasting to ensure that you're meeting your nutritional needs, maintaining energy levels, and supporting overall well-being. Here are some key signals to pay attention to and how to respond to them:

1. *Hunger:* Pay attention to your body's hunger cues and eat when you feel genuinely hungry. While fasting, it's normal to experience mild hunger pangs, especially during the initial adjustment period.

However, if you're experiencing persistent or severe hunger, it may be a sign that you need to adjust your fasting schedule or meal timing to better align with your body's needs. Choose nutrient-dense foods to help satisfy hunger and provide sustained energy throughout the fasting period.

2. *Energy Levels:* Notice how your energy levels fluctuate throughout the day and adjust your activities accordingly. If you're feeling low on energy or fatigued, it may be a sign that you need to rest or refuel with nourishing foods. Prioritize activities that align with your energy levels, and avoid pushing yourself too hard during fasting periods.

3. *Thirst:* Stay hydrated by drinking plenty of water throughout the day and listen to your body's signals for thirst. Dehydration can mimic feelings of hunger, so it's essential to replenish fluids regularly, especially during fasting periods. Aim to drink at least 8-10 glasses of water per day, and consider incorporating hydrating beverages like herbal tea or infused water for added flavor and hydration.

4. *Digestive Health:* Pay attention to how your body responds to different foods and adjust your diet accordingly to support digestive health. If you're experiencing digestive discomfort or bloating, it may be a sign that certain foods don't agree with you. Consider experimenting with your meal composition and timing to find what works best for your body and promotes optimal digestion.

5. *Mood and Well-being:* Notice how your mood and overall well-being are affected by fasting and adjust your routine accordingly. If you're feeling irritable, anxious, or low in mood, it may be a sign that you need to prioritize self-care practices like mindfulness, relaxation, or social connection. Listen to your body's signals for rest and relaxation, and make time for activities that promote emotional well-being during fasting periods.

6.2 Incorporating Exercise for Optimal Results

Incorporating exercise into your intermittent fasting routine can enhance the effectiveness of your fasting regimen and help you achieve optimal results in terms of weight loss, metabolic health, and overall well-being. Here are some key considerations for incorporating exercise while fasting:

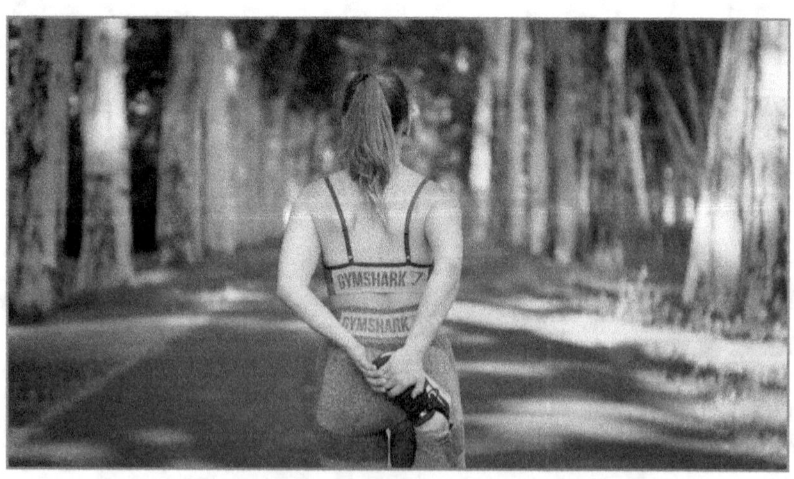

1. *Timing:* Experiment with different timing strategies to find the best time to exercise within your fasting window. Some people prefer to exercise in a fasted state, such as first thing in the morning before breaking their fast, while others may prefer to exercise during their eating window to fuel their workouts. Listen to your body and choose a timing that aligns with your energy levels and preferences.

2. *Types of Exercise:* Incorporate a combination of cardiovascular exercise, strength training, and flexibility exercises to achieve a well-rounded fitness routine. Cardiovascular activities like walking, running, cycling, or swimming can help burn calories and improve cardiovascular health. Strength training exercises like weightlifting or bodyweight exercises can help build muscle mass and boost metabolism. Flexibility exercises like yoga or stretching can improve mobility and reduce the risk of injury.

3. *Intensity:* Adjust the intensity of your workouts based on your fitness level, energy levels, and fasting status. While high-intensity workouts can be effective for calorie burning and improving fitness, they may be more challenging to perform in a fasted state. Consider integrating a mix of moderate-intensity and high-intensity workouts to balance energy expenditure and recovery.

4. *Hydration and Nutrition:* Stay hydrated before, during, and after exercise by drinking plenty of water, especially during fasting periods. If you're exercising in a fasted state, consider consuming a small snack or beverage containing carbohydrates and electrolytes to help sustain energy levels and prevent dehydration. After exercising, prioritize refueling with nutrient-rich foods to support muscle recovery and replenish glycogen stores.

5. *Listen to Your Body:* Pay attention to how your body responds to exercise while fasting and adjust your routine accordingly, this cannot be overemphasized. If you're experiencing excessive fatigue, dizziness, or other negative side effects, it may be a sign that you need to modify your exercise intensity or timing. Listen to your body's cues and make changes as needed to support your overall well-being.

6.3 Tracking Your Progress and Adjusting Strategies

Tracking your progress and adjusting strategies is crucial for achieving success with intermittent fasting and reaching your health and wellness goals. By monitoring key metrics and making informed adjustments to your fasting regimen, you can optimize your results and maintain long-term adherence to your fasting routine.

Here's how to effectively track your progress and make necessary adjustments:

1. Establish Clear Goals: Begin by setting clear, realistic goals for your intermittent fasting journey. Whether your objectives include weight loss, improved metabolic health, increased energy levels, or other health-related outcomes, having specific goals will help you stay focused and motivated throughout the process.

2. Track Key Metrics: Identify key metrics to track your progress and measure the effectiveness of your fasting regimen. Common metrics to monitor may include weight, body measurements, body fat percentage, fasting blood glucose levels, energy levels, mood, and overall well-being. Use a journal, spreadsheet, or tracking app to record these metrics regularly.

3. Monitor Changes: Consistently monitor changes in your tracked metrics over time to assess the impact of intermittent fasting on your health and wellness. Pay attention to trends and patterns in your data, noting any fluctuations or trends that may indicate progress or areas for improvement.

4. Experiment with Strategies: Be open to experimenting with different fasting protocols, meal timings, nutrient ratios, and exercise routines to find what works best for your body. Consider trying alternate-day fasting, time-restricted eating, or different fasting windows to see how your body responds. Experiment with meal composition, portion sizes, and food choices to optimize satiety and nutritional balance.

5. *Adjust as Needed:* Based on your progress and feedback from your body, make informed adjustments to your fasting regimen to optimize results. If you're not seeing the desired outcomes or experiencing negative side effects, consider tweaking your fasting schedule, meal timing, or nutrient intake. Consult with a healthcare professional or registered dietitian for personalized guidance and support.

6. *Celebrate Milestones:* Celebrate your achievements and milestones along the way to keep yourself motivated and engaged with your intermittent fasting journey. Whether it's reaching a weight loss goal, improving metabolic markers, or experiencing increased energy levels, acknowledge and celebrate your progress to maintain momentum and stay committed to your goals.

7. *Stay Consistent:* Consistency is key to seeing long-term results with intermittent fasting. Stay committed to your fasting regimen and lifestyle changes, even during periods of setbacks or challenges. Remember that progress takes

time, and stay patient and persistent in your efforts to achieve your health and wellness goals.

CHAPTER 7

Exploring Advanced Techniques

7.1 Combining Intermittent Fasting with Other Diets

Combining intermittent fasting with other diets can be an effective approach to enhance weight loss, improve metabolic health, and achieve overall well-being. By integrating fasting principles with various dietary patterns, individuals can tailor their eating habits to suit their preferences, lifestyle, and health goals. Here's how to combine intermittent fasting with popular diets for optimal results:

1. *Ketogenic Diet (Keto):* The ketogenic diet focuses on consuming high-fat, moderate-protein, and low-carbohydrate foods to induce a state of ketosis, where the body burns fat for fuel instead of carbohydrates.

Combining intermittent fasting with the keto diet can enhance fat burning and promote weight loss. Consider following a time-restricted eating pattern, such as fasting for 16 hours and eating within an 8-hour window, while adhering to keto-friendly foods during eating periods. This can help increase fat oxidation and support ketone production, leading to greater fat loss and metabolic benefits.

2. *Mediterranean Diet:* The Mediterranean diet emphasizes whole, minimally processed foods such as fruits, vegetables, whole grains, legumes, nuts, seeds, and olive oil, along with moderate consumption of fish, poultry, and dairy products.

Combining intermittent fasting with the Mediterranean diet can enhance the diet's health-promoting effects and improve weight management. Try incorporating a fasting protocol, such as alternate-day fasting or time-restricted eating, while following Mediterranean-style meals during eating periods. This can help regulate appetite, improve insulin sensitivity, and reduce inflammation, leading to better overall health outcomes.

3.Paleo Diet: The paleo diet focuses on consuming foods that were available to our hunter-gatherer ancestors, such as lean meats, fish, fruits, vegetables, nuts, and seeds, while excluding processed foods, grains, legumes, and dairy products.

Combining intermittent fasting with the paleo diet can enhance fat loss, improve metabolic health, and support overall well-being. Consider following a fasting protocol, such as the 16/8 method or intermittent fasting on alternate days, while adhering to paleo-friendly foods during eating periods. This can help regulate blood sugar levels, promote fat burning, and optimize nutrient intake, leading to improved health outcomes.

4.*Plant-Based Diet:* A plant-based diet focuses on consuming primarily whole, plant-based foods such as fruits, vegetables, grains, legumes, nuts, and seeds, while minimizing or eliminating animal products.

Combining intermittent fasting with a plant-based diet can enhance weight loss, improve metabolic health, and reduce inflammation. Try incorporating a fasting protocol, such as time-restricted eating or intermittent fasting on alternate days, while following plant-based meals during eating periods. This can help increase fat oxidation, support cellular repair processes, and promote overall health and longevity.

6. *Low-Carb Diet:* A low-carb diet focuses on reducing carbohydrate intake while increasing consumption of protein and healthy fats. Combining intermittent fasting with a low-carb diet can enhance fat burning, improve insulin sensitivity, and support weight loss.

Consider following a fasting protocol, such as time-restricted eating or intermittent fasting on alternate days, while adhering to low-carb foods during eating periods. This can help optimize fat metabolism, regulate blood sugar levels, and promote sustainable weight loss over time.

7.2 Fasting for Mental Clarity and Focus

Fasting for mental clarity and focus has gained attention as a potential way to enhance cognitive function, improve productivity, and support overall brain health.

While much of the research on fasting has focused on its effects on weight loss and metabolic health, emerging evidence suggests that fasting may also have profound benefits for the brain. Here's how fasting can impact mental clarity and focus:

1. Enhanced Brain Function: Fasting triggers a metabolic switch in the body, shifting from glucose metabolism to ketone metabolism during periods of fasting. Ketones, which are produced from the breakdown of fats, serve as an alternative fuel source for the brain when glucose levels are low.

This metabolic shift has been associated with improved cognitive function, enhanced memory, and increased mental clarity. By providing the brain with a readily available source of energy, fasting may support optimal brain function and cognitive performance.

2. *Neuroprotection:* Fasting has been shown to activate various cellular pathways and molecular mechanisms that promote brain health and protect against neurodegenerative diseases. Studies have demonstrated that fasting can stimulate the production of brain-derived neurotrophic factor (BDNF), a protein that plays a key role in neuroplasticity, neuronal growth, and synaptic function.

Increased levels of BDNF have been linked to improved cognitive function, enhanced memory formation, and reduced risk of neurodegenerative disorders such as Alzheimer's disease and Parkinson's disease.

3. *Reduced Inflammation:* Chronic inflammation has been implicated in the development of cognitive decline and neurological disorders. Fasting has been shown to reduce inflammation in the body by suppressing pro-inflammatory cytokines and activating anti-inflammatory pathways.

By reducing systemic inflammation, fasting may help protect against neuroinflammation and support brain health. This anti-inflammatory effect of fasting may contribute to improved mental clarity, focus, and overall cognitive function.

4. Autophagy: Fasting stimulates a process known as autophagy, which is the body's natural mechanism for cellular repair and recycling. During fasting, cells undergo autophagy to remove damaged or dysfunctional components and promote cellular renewal.

This process has been shown to have neuroprotective effects and may help clear out toxic proteins and aggregates that accumulate in the brain with age. By promoting autophagy, fasting may support brain health, improve cognitive function, and enhance mental clarity and focus.

6. *Hormonal Balance:* Fasting can also impact hormone levels in the body, including hormones that influence brain function and cognitive performance. For example, fasting has been shown to increase levels of norepinephrine and dopamine, neurotransmitters that play key roles in attention, motivation, and executive function.

Additionally, fasting can improve insulin sensitivity and regulate blood sugar levels, which are important for brain health and cognitive function. By promoting hormonal balance, fasting may support mental clarity, focus, and overall brain function.

7.3 Intermittent Fasting for Long-Term Health and Longevity

Intermittent fasting has garnered attention not only for its potential to aid in weight loss but also for its profound impact on long-term health and longevity.

Emerging research suggests that intermittent fasting may offer a range of benefits that can contribute to overall well-being and extend lifespan. Here's how intermittent fasting can promote long-term health and longevity:

1. *Enhanced Metabolic Health:* Intermittent fasting has been shown to improve various markers of metabolic health, including insulin sensitivity, blood sugar control, and lipid levels.

By promoting more efficient energy utilization and metabolic flexibility, intermittent fasting may help reduce the risk of metabolic diseases such as type 2 diabetes, cardiovascular disease, and obesity. Improved metabolic health is associated with a lower risk of chronic diseases and may contribute to a longer and healthier life.

2. *Cellular Repair and Regeneration:* Fasting triggers a process called autophagy, which is the body's natural

mechanism for cellular repair and regeneration. During fasting, cells undergo autophagy to remove damaged or dysfunctional components and promote cellular renewal. This process has been linked to a range of health benefits, including reduced inflammation, improved immune function, and enhanced cellular longevity. By promoting autophagy, intermittent fasting may help protect against age-related decline and support overall health and longevity.

3. *Reduction of Chronic Inflammation:* Chronic inflammation is a key driver of aging and age-related diseases. Intermittent fasting has been shown to reduce systemic inflammation by suppressing pro-inflammatory cytokines and activating anti-inflammatory pathways.

By reducing inflammation in the body, intermittent fasting may help prevent or mitigate the development of chronic diseases associated with aging, such as cardiovascular disease, neurodegenerative disorders, and cancer. Lower levels of inflammation are associated with improved healthspan and increased longevity.

3. *Protection Against Age-Related Cognitive Decline:* Intermittent fasting has been shown to support brain health and protect against age-related cognitive decline. Fasting stimulates the production of brain-derived

neurotrophic factor (BDNF), a protein that promotes neuronal growth, synaptic plasticity, and cognitive function.

Increased levels of BDNF have been linked to improved memory, learning, and cognitive resilience against neurodegenerative diseases such as Alzheimer's and Parkinson's disease. By promoting brain health, intermittent fasting may help preserve cognitive function and promote longevity.

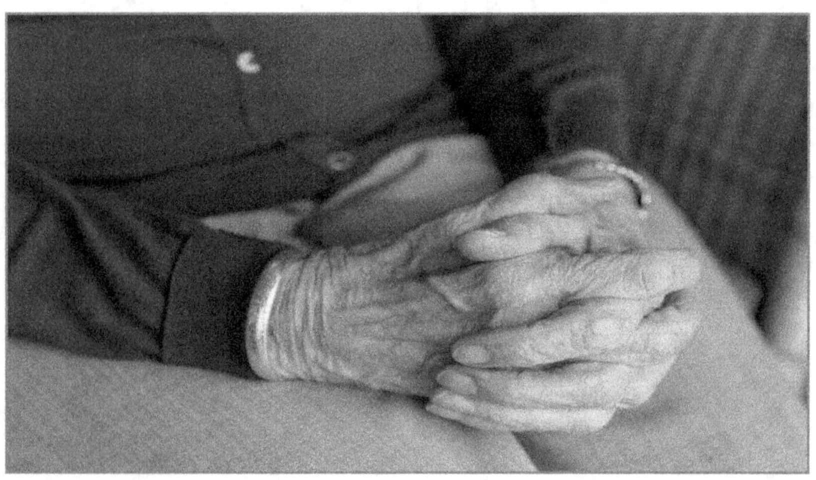

4. Stress Resistance and Hormesis: Intermittent fasting induces a mild stress response in the body, which activates adaptive cellular pathways that promote resilience and longevity. This phenomenon, known as hormesis, involves exposing the body to moderate stressors that trigger protective responses and enhance stress resistance.

By activating stress-responsive pathways such as sirtuins, FOXO proteins, and AMPK, intermittent fasting may help increase cellular resilience, improve mitochondrial function, and extend lifespan.

6. *Maintenance of Healthy Weight:* Maintaining a healthy weight is a key factor in promoting longevity and reducing the risk of obesity-related diseases. Intermittent fasting can be an effective strategy for weight management by promoting fat loss, preserving lean muscle mass, and regulating appetite. By reducing excess body fat and improving metabolic health, intermittent fasting may help prevent obesity-related complications and promote longevity.

Conclusion

Celebrating Your Intermittent Fasting Success

Celebrating your intermittent fasting success is an important aspect of maintaining motivation, staying committed to your goals, and recognizing your achievements along the way. Here are some ways to celebrate your intermittent fasting success:

1. Set Milestones: Break down your long-term goals into smaller, achievable milestones. Celebrate each milestone you reach, whether it's completing your first week of intermittent fasting, reaching a specific weight loss target, or noticing improvements in your energy levels or overall well-being.

2. Reward Yourself: Treat yourself to a non-food reward when you achieve a significant milestone or accomplish a specific goal. Whether it's buying yourself a new outfit, booking a spa day, or indulging in a favorite hobby, rewarding yourself for your hard work and dedication can help reinforce positive behavior and motivate you to keep going.

3. *Share Your Success:* Share your intermittent fasting success with friends, family, or a supportive community. Celebrate your achievements publicly by posting about them on social media, joining an online forum or support group, or simply sharing your progress with loved ones. Celebrating your success with others can help boost your confidence, inspire others to pursue their own health goals, and reinforce your commitment to intermittent fasting.

4. *Reflect on Your Journey:* Take time to reflect on how far you've come since starting your intermittent fasting journey. Consider keeping a journal to document your progress, challenges, and successes along the way. Reflecting on your journey can help you appreciate your accomplishments, learn from setbacks, and stay motivated to continue pursuing your health and wellness goals.

5. *Practice Gratitude:* Cultivate a sense of gratitude for the progress you've made and the positive changes you've experienced as a result of intermittent fasting. Take a moment each day to acknowledge and appreciate the small victories, whether it's feeling more energized, sleeping better, or simply feeling proud of yourself for sticking to your fasting regimen. Practicing gratitude can help shift your mindset toward positivity and enhance your overall well-being.

The Continued Journey to Optimal Health

The journey to optimal health is a continuous and evolving process that extends beyond achieving specific goals or milestones. It involves making sustainable lifestyle changes, prioritizing self-care, and embracing a holistic approach to well-being. Here's how to continue your journey to optimal health:

1. *Consistency and Persistence:* Stay committed to your health goals and maintain consistency in your habits and routines. Incorporate healthy behaviors into your daily life, such as eating nutritious foods, staying active, getting enough sleep, managing stress, and practicing self-care. Consistent efforts over time are key to achieving and maintaining optimal health.

2. *Lifelong Learning:* Keep an open mind and continue to educate yourself about health and wellness topics. Stay informed about the latest research, trends, and best practices in nutrition, exercise, mindfulness, and other areas of well-being. Seek out reputable sources of information and be willing to adapt your approach based on new evidence and insights.

3. *Listening to Your Body:* Pay attention to your body's signals and adjust your habits and behaviors accordingly. Tune in to how different foods, activities, and lifestyle

choices make you feel physically, mentally, and emotionally. Listen to your body's cues for hunger, thirst, fatigue, and stress, and respond with compassion and self-care.

4. *Setting New Goals:* Continuously challenge yourself to set new health goals and aspirations. Whether it's improving your fitness level, trying new healthy recipes, reducing stress, or prioritizing self-care, set specific, measurable, and achievable goals that align with your values and priorities. Celebrate your progress along the way and stay motivated by focusing on the positive changes you're making.

5. *Seeking Support:* Surround yourself with a supportive network of family, friends, and health professionals who can cheer you on, provide encouragement, and offer guidance when needed. Share your health goals and aspirations with others, and don't hesitate to ask for help or support when facing challenges or setbacks. Together, you can inspire and empower each other to pursue optimal health and well-being.

6. *Embracing Balance:* Strive for balance in all aspects of your life, including diet, exercise, work, relationships, and leisure activities. Avoid extremes or rigid rules that may lead to feelings of deprivation, guilt, or burnout. Instead,

aim for a flexible and sustainable approach that allows you to enjoy life while also prioritizing your health and well-being.

By staying committed to your health goals, listening to your body, seeking support, and embracing a holistic approach to well-being, you can continue to thrive and live your best life at every stage of your journey.

Appendix

Nutrient-Rich Food List

Adding nutrient-rich foods into your diet is essential for supporting overall health, optimizing energy levels, and promoting well-being. Here's a comprehensive list of nutrient-rich foods to include in your meals:

Vegetables:

- Leafy greens (spinach, kale, Swiss chard, arugula)

- Cruciferous vegetables (broccoli, cauliflower, Brussels sprouts)

- Colorful vegetables (bell peppers, carrots, tomatoes, sweet potatoes)

- Allium vegetables (garlic, onions, leeks)

- Root vegetables (beets, turnips, radishes)

Fruits:

- Berries (blueberries, strawberries, raspberries)

- Citrus fruits (oranges, lemons, grapefruits)

- Apples

- Bananas

- Kiwi

- Mangoes

- Pineapple

- Avocado

Whole Grains:

- Quinoa

- Brown rice

- Oats

- Barley

- Bulgur

- Farro

- Whole wheat pasta

- Whole grain bread

Protein Sources:

- Lean meats (chicken breast, turkey breast, lean cuts of beef or pork)

- Fish (salmon, tuna, mackerel, trout)

- Eggs

- Legumes (beans, lentils, chickpeas)

- Tofu

- Tempeh

- Edamame

Dairy and Dairy Alternatives:

- Greek yogurt

- Cottage cheese

- Skim or low-fat milk

- Plant-based milk (almond milk, soy milk, coconut milk)

- Cheese (in moderation)

- Nuts and Seeds:

- Almonds

- Walnuts

- Cashews

- Pistachios

- Chia seeds

- Flaxseeds

- Pumpkin seeds

- Sunflower seeds

Healthy Fats:

- Olive oil

- Avocado oil

- Coconut oil

- Fatty fish (salmon, sardines, trout)

- Nuts and seeds

- Avocado

Herbs and Spices:

- Turmeric

- Ginger

- Cinnamon

- Garlic

- Basil

- Rosemary

- Thyme

- Parsley

Aim to include a colorful array of fruits and vegetables, lean protein sources, whole grains, and healthy fats in your meals to support your overall nutrition and vitality.

A 30-Day Customized Balanced Meal Plan For The 16/8 Method Of Intermittent Fasting

Day 1:

12:00 PM (First Meal): Scrambled eggs with spinach and feta cheese, served with whole grain toast

3:00 PM (Second Meal): Grilled chicken salad with mixed greens, cherry tomatoes, cucumbers, and balsamic vinaigrette

7:00 PM (Last Meal): Baked salmon with quinoa and roasted vegetables

Day 2:

12:00 PM (First Meal): Greek yogurt with mixed berries and a drizzle of honey

3:00 PM (Second Meal): Turkey and avocado wrap with whole grain tortilla, lettuce, tomato, and mustard

7:00 PM (Last Meal): Stir-fried tofu with broccoli, bell peppers, and brown rice

Day 3:

12:00 PM (First Meal): Oatmeal topped with sliced bananas, almonds, and a sprinkle of cinnamon

3:00 PM (Second Meal): Quinoa salad with mixed greens, chickpeas, cucumbers, cherry tomatoes, and lemon-tahini dressing

7:00 PM (Last Meal): Grilled shrimp skewers with quinoa pilaf and grilled asparagus

Days 4-6:

12:00 PM (First Meal): Smoothie made with spinach, banana, almond milk, and protein powder

3:00 PM (Second Meal): Lentil soup with a side salad

7:00 PM (Last Meal): Baked chicken breast with sweet potato mash and steamed green beans

Days 7-9:

12:00 PM (First Meal): Chia seed pudding with sliced strawberries and almonds

3:00 PM (Second Meal): Turkey chili with beans, served with a side of Greek yogurt and chopped cilantro

7:00 PM (Last Meal): Grilled salmon with quinoa salad and steamed broccoli

Continue with this pattern, ensuring to include a variety of nutrient-rich foods, until you complete the 30-day plan. Adjust portion sizes and meal timings according to your individual needs and preferences.

30-Day Customized Balanced Meal Plan For The 5:2 Diet:

Day 1 (Fasting Day):

Breakfast: Black coffee or herbal tea (0 calories)

Lunch: Vegetable soup (200 calories)

Dinner: Baked salmon with steamed broccoli (300 calories)

Day 2 (Feeding Day):

Breakfast: Greek yogurt with mixed berries and a sprinkle of granola (250 calories)

Lunch: Turkey and avocado wrap with whole grain tortilla (350 calories)

Dinner: Grilled chicken breast with quinoa and roasted vegetables (400 calories)

Day 3 (Fasting Day):

Breakfast: Green tea (0 calories)

Lunch: Lentil soup (200 calories)

Dinner: Grilled tofu with stir-fried vegetables (300 calories)

Days 4-6: Repeat the meal plan from Day 2

Days 7-9: Repeat the meal plan from Day 3

Days 10-12:

Fasting Day: Vegetable broth (50 calories)

Feeding Day:

Breakfast: Smoothie made with spinach, banana, almond milk, and protein powder (250 calories)

Lunch: Quinoa salad with mixed greens, chickpeas, cucumbers, and lemon-tahini dressing (350 calories)

Dinner: Baked cod with roasted sweet potatoes and asparagus (400 calories)

Continue rotating through different meal options for the remaining days of the 30-day plan, ensuring that fasting days are limited to 500-600 calories for women and 600-800 calories for men, while feeding days provide balanced nutrition from whole, minimally processed foods.

30-Day Customized Balanced Meal Plan For The OMAD (One Meal a Day) Approach:

Day 1:

Dinner: Grilled chicken breast with quinoa pilaf and roasted vegetables

Day 2:

Dinner: Baked salmon with sweet potato mash and steamed broccoli

Day 3:

Dinner: Stir-fried tofu with mixed vegetables and brown rice

Day 4:

Dinner: Turkey chili with beans, served with a side salad

Day 5:

Dinner: Beef stir-fry with bell peppers, onions, and snow peas over cauliflower rice

Day 6:

Dinner: Spaghetti squash with marinara sauce, lean ground turkey, and a side of garlic bread

Day 7:

Dinner: Grilled shrimp skewers with quinoa salad and grilled asparagus

Days 8-14:

Repeat the meal plan from Day 1-7

Days 15-21:

Repeat the meal plan from Day 1-7

Days 22-28:

Repeat the meal plan from Day 1-7

Days 29-30:

Dinner: Homemade vegetable curry with chickpeas, served over brown rice

 It's important to ensure that your one meal provides all the essential nutrients your body needs for optimal health and well-being.

A 30-Day Customized Balanced Meal Plan For Alternate Day Fasting:

Day 1 (Feeding Day):

Breakfast: Greek yogurt with mixed berries and a sprinkle of granola

Lunch: Turkey and avocado wrap with whole grain tortilla

Dinner: Grilled salmon with quinoa pilaf and roasted vegetables

Day 2 (Fasting Day):

Breakfast: Green tea

Lunch: Vegetable soup

Dinner: Baked chicken breast with steamed broccoli

Day 3 (Feeding Day):

Breakfast: Oatmeal topped with sliced bananas and almonds

Lunch: Lentil salad with mixed greens, cherry tomatoes, and balsamic vinaigrette

Dinner: Stir-fried tofu with brown rice and mixed vegetables

Days 4-6:

Feeding Day: Repeat the meal plan from Day 1

Fasting Day: Repeat the meal plan from Day 2

Days 7-9:

Feeding Day: Repeat the meal plan from Day 3

Fasting Day: Repeat the meal plan from Day 2

Days 10-12:

Feeding Day: Smoothie made with spinach, banana, almond milk, and protein powder for breakfast; Grilled chicken salad for lunch; Baked cod with quinoa and roasted vegetables for dinner

Fasting Day: Repeat the meal plan from Day 2

Continue rotating through different meal options for the remaining days of the 30-day plan, ensuring that fasting days are limited to 500-600 calories for women and 600-800 calories for men, while feeding days provide balanced nutrition from whole, minimally processed foods.

Remember to stay hydrated throughout the fasting period and listen to your body's hunger cues. Consult with a healthcare professional before starting any new diet plan, especially if you have underlying health conditions or dietary restrictions.

About the Author

Sarah Carsen, a seasoned nutritionist and passionate wellness advocate, brings over a decade of expertise to her latest endeavor. With a focus on digestive wellness and holistic health, she is renowned for offering tailored guidance and effective strategies.

Her latest masterpiece, *"Intermittent Fasting for Beginners: The Ultimate Guide to Effortless Weight Loss and Optimal Health,"* epitomizes her commitment to empowering individuals towards better health and vitality. In this comprehensive guide, Sarah leverages her wealth of knowledge to demystify intermittent fasting and unveil its Game-changing potential.

Through her meticulous approach and compassionate guidance, she inspires readers to embark on a journey towards sustainable weight loss and enhanced well-being. With Sarah's expertise as a trusted companion, individuals are empowered to make lasting, positive changes for their health and vitality.